Neuroplasticity Of The Brain

How To Overhaul Your Personality, Kill Bad Habits And Achieve Your Goals Using The New Science Of The Brain

Andreas Senkbeil

Andreas Senkbeil

© Copyright 2016 by Andreas Senkbeil - All rights reserved.

This document is geared towards providing exact and reliable information in regards to the topic and issue covered. The publication is sold with the idea that the publisher is not required to render accounting, officially permitted, or otherwise, qualified services. If advice is necessary, legal or professional, a practiced individual in the profession should be ordered.

- From a Declaration of Principles which was accepted and approved equally by a Committee of the American Bar Association and a Committee of Publishers and Associations.

In no way is it legal to reproduce, duplicate, or transmit any part of this document in either electronic means or in printed format. Recording of this publication is strictly prohibited and any storage of this document is not allowed unless with written permission from the publisher. All rights reserved.

The information provided herein is stated to be truthful and consistent, in that any liability, in terms of inattention or otherwise, by any usage or abuse of any policies, processes, or directions contained within is the solitary and utter responsibility of the recipient reader. Under no circumstances will any legal responsibility or blame be held against the publisher for any reparation, damages, or monetary loss due to the information herein, either directly or indirectly.

Respective authors own all copyrights not held by the publisher.

Neuroplasticity Of The Brain

The information herein is offered for informational purposes solely, and is universal as so. The presentation of the information is without contract or any type of guarantee assurance.

The trademarks that are used are without any consent, and the publication of the trademark is without permission or backing by the trademark owner. All trademarks and brands within this book are for clarifying purposes only and are the owned by the owners themselves, not affiliated with this document

Andreas Senkbeil

TABLE OF CONTENT

Chapter 1: What Is Neuroplasticity? — 1

Chapter 2: Overhaul Your Attitude And Shape A More Positive Mind — 12

Chapter 3: Enliven Your Learning — 22

Chapter 4: Go For Your Goals — 34

Conclusion: Where To Go From Here — 43

Chapter 1: What Is Neuroplasticity?

What you will learn in this book will change your life

You are about to embark on a journey into the exciting world of neuroplasticity. In this chapter, you will learn what "neuroplasticity" means, along with some basic brain terminology that will help you understand what is really going on inside your brain when you learn a new skill or expand your knowledge base. You will be taken on a brief tour of the exciting research that psychologists have carried out which proves neuroplasticity to be an exciting phenomenon that has been observed in many different groups across dozens of scientific studies. You will then learn exactly how you can make the most of these findings in improving your everyday life, capacity for learning, and even in helping regulate your mood. You will also understand why your first concern should be fixing your diet and sleep patterns before you can take full advantage of your wonderfully plastic brain.

What is "neuroplasticity"?

At its most basic, the term " neuroplasticity " refers to the brain"s ability to change. Our brains are not lumps of inert gray matter sitting in our skulls. They are dynamic organs that continue developing from the first weeks of life to the moment of death. Every time you interact with your surroundings or engage in any particular behaviour, the relevant pathways are reinforced within your brain. The key message to take from this book is as follows: When you change the way you behave and the way you think, you can make huge leaps forward in developing your potential as a human being. The science of neuroplasticity has enabled academics, doctors and everyone interested in self-development to take a more optimistic view of human potential for growth and change at any age. So if you want to start leading a happier, more productive life – and who doesn"t?! – then learning about neuroplasticity and its applications is a great place to start.

Brain 101 – the basics

To fully appreciate neuroplasticity, it"s important that you understand a few basic concepts and terms. Don"t worry – there aren"t too many! However, to get the most from this book, there are a few pieces of background information you need to know.

First of all, it"s helpful to know a little bit about the way in which your brain is structured. When you think of a brain, you probably imagine the outer layer – the part that appears gray and wrinkled. The scientific name for this area of the brain is the cerebrum. It is divided in two halves, known as the cerebral hemispheres. Underneath the external gray area (also known as "gray matter") there is a white layer known as "white matter." Most scientists agree that it is the cerebrum that makes us human. It grants us the capability to engage in reflection, learning, and other conscious mental processes. The cerebrum tends to be well-developed (with more wrinkles) in animal species known for their intelligence, such as dolphins, elephants and non-human primates such as chimpanzees.

How your brain is structured

Within the cerebrum, we have four regions or lobes. They are as follows:

Frontal Lobe: This helps us make decisions and plans. It

lets us look into the future, delay gratification, and behave in a responsible manner. These do not finish developing until our twenties, which goes some way in explaining why children and adolescents typically find it difficult to look far into the future and make good long-term decisions.
Parietal Lobe: This helps us pay attention to our surroundings and is also responsible for spatial awareness. Your parietal lobe helps you navigate a new place, catch a ball, and notice what something feels like.

Temporal Lobe: This allows us to comprehend language, to make sense of what we hear, and to draw on existing auditory memories.

Occipital Lobe: This helps us process and make use of visual information. To fully appreciate what is going on in the world around you, not only do you need a pair of working eyes but you also need to be able to make sense of this sensory information. The occipital lobe allows you to do just that.

The beauty of brain cells

There are many different types of cell that make up the human brain, but arguably the most important kind to note when talking about neuroplasticity are neurons. These cells are responsible for transmitting information throughout the brain using chemical and electrical signals. There are around 86 billion neurons in the average human brain. Every neuron is capable of making around 10,000 connections with other neurons. That represents a huge number of potential connections! Neurons start developing within the first month of human life. An embryo develops 250,000 neurons per minute. This rapid neuronal growth is known as neurogenesis. Previously it was believed that neurogenesis ended in early childhood, but it turns out that our brains can generate new neurons throughout our lifetimes.

Between our neurons we have synapses, which are simply tiny gaps which allow two or more neurons to pass on these chemical or electrical signals. At birth we have approximately 2,500 synapses, which then increases to 15,000 at three years of age.

A change in perspective – how scientists have shifted their theories of neuroplasticity

As previously noted, the concept of neuroplasticity is so exciting because for centuries it was thought that the human brain could not change once a person had reached physical maturity. So why did scientists used to believe that the brain was fixed, a machine that wasn"t capable of expansion or growth?

Firstly, people with brain damage seldom appeared to recover from their injuries. For example, neurologist Paul Broca observed that most people with damage to Broca"s area (a part of the brain located in the frontal lobe) suffered an impairment in their ability to produce speech, and they seldom regained these abilities. As science uncovered more links between particular brain areas and functions, the idea that we rely on specific brain areas for various cognitive abilities become more widespread. Secondly, it has only been in the past few decades that we have been able to see how the brain actually works in real time. Human and animal experiments have shown the brain"s ability to form new connections between neurons in response to actions and intentional thought patterns. We now have access to technology that can monitor connections between, and the activity of, individual neurons. We can scan human and animal brains as they undertake various cognitive tasks, and we can take images on a regular basis that allows us to understand the relationship between behavioral change and neuronal change.

Neuroplasticity in action

A major turning point in the science of neuroplasticity arose from the discovery that people who suffer from brain damage can and do recover some of their lost abilities. It turns out that when an area of the brain usually responsible for a particular function is damaged, with appropriate training another part of the brain can leap in and take over. In addition, damaged areas of the brain can be retrained and to some extent restored if an appropriate programme of ongoing rehabilitation is followed. For example, when someone suffers from a stroke (an event in which a blood clot prevents the delivery of oxygen to one or more areas of the brain), they will typically be left with difficulties in speaking and movement on one side of their body. In order to let the patient regain the use of their limbs and speech capacity, they will be asked to follow a comprehensive rehabilitation programme. At the heart of every well-structured recovery regimen is a series of exercises that are repeated for hours over the course of days, weeks, months or even years. The logic is simple – in order to help the damaged areas of the brain heal, it is necessary to encourage new connections to develop between existing neurons and also to encourage neurogenesis. In this way, the old neuronal networks will be reactivated and the patient will regain some of their lost abilities.

Research with healthy volunteers has shown that when we lose the ability to see, our other senses become heightened in response. Scientists from the University of Montreal have shown that when we are deprived of our sense of sight for as little as 90 minutes, we are better at being able to locate sounds in space. Furthermore, people who are truly blind often demonstrate greater capabilities in this respect than those who are sighted. This is yet more evidence suggesting that our brains can change rapidly in response to various circumstances and external stimulation. The average human brain has the astonishing ability to devote more or less resources to specific functions depending on the situation.

Why did our brains evolve to be plastic?

Human beings are without doubt one of the most successful species on Earth. Our capacity for language, complex thought and the creation of culture has resulted in our domination (for better or worse) over almost the entire planet. One of the key factors behind this success is the way in which our brains can adapt to whatever new challenges we face. This explains why humans have managed to carve out a niche for themselves in almost every environment on earth. Whether we are living on a frozen tundra or in tropical rainforests, every human society has managed to devise ways of coping with the challenges and perils facing them. Over the many tens of thousands of years underlying human evolution, those who have been best able to adapt – i.e., those with the most plastic brains – have been most likely to thrive in even harsh environments, and pass on this adaptability to their offspring.

What do taxi drivers, musicians and jugglers have in common?

Psychologists have also been able to demonstrate neuroplasticity using brain scanning methods such as Magnetic Resonance Imaging (known as MRI). One of the most famous studies in neuroplasticity to date featured London taxi drivers. Becoming a driver in England"s capital is not easy – in order to be successful, you need to develop a comprehensive working knowledge of the city"s layout. This understanding is referred to, fittingly enough, as "The Knowledge," and the test they must pass in order to obtain their full licence is known as "The Knowledge Test." The average wannabe-driver must spend years learning how to navigate the 25,000 streets that lie within a six-mile radius of Charing Cross at the heart of London. This specialized skill has made London taxi drivers especially worthy of study. Researchers Eleanor Maguire and Katherine Woollett, based at University College London, decided to investigate whether the act of learning "The Knowledge" left an impression – quite literally – on drivers" brains. They scanned the brains of 79 trainee drivers over the course of several years, using MRI technology to monitor any brain changes triggered by their intensive course of study. The process of preparing for the final test is so demanding that in the end, only 39 of the 79 trainees ended up passing the test. In the end, the researchers ended up tracking the progress of three groups – those that trained to be a taxi driver and passed the test, those that trained but didn"t pass, and a control group of people who never undertook any training in the first place. Their findings were remarkable. In the trainee drivers who learned the city layout and passed the tests, the hippocampus – a part of the brain responsible for spatial learning – grew in size. This effect was not observed in either the control group or those who had tried to acquire "The Knowledge" but later failed the test. Furthermore, ongoing research showed that the longer a person works as a taxi driver, the larger their hippocampus will grow. This is an excellent example of how, with the right attitude and intention, you can literally shape your brain by exposing yourself to new knowledge and experiences. Musicians have also contributed to the science of neuroplasticity. A research review published in the journal *Frontiers in Psychology* suggests that musical training changes brain structure and function. It seems likely that the brains of people who play a musical instrument on a regular basis become more adept at combining auditory input and enacting motor movements in response to these stimuli. When you read music and play an instrument at the same time, your brain is forced to integrate visual and auditory information. Therefore, it seems likely that musical training encourages what is known as "audio-visual integration." With increased practice and dedication to playing a musical instrument, the brain becomes even better at this kind of cognitive processing. Research has also focused on the effects of short-term training on specific brain areas. For example, a paper published in *PLoS One* described a study in which healthy adult volunteers were trained how to juggle. Twenty people were trained to juggle with three balls before having their brains scanned 7, 14 and 35 days later. Within a week of regular juggling practice, the volunteers" occipital lobes had changed. Specifically, an area known as V5 – which is responsible for detecting objects in space, a skill important for successful throwing and catching juggling balls – had become denser. This was a simple, clear-cut example of how the human brain changes as a direct response to input and effort. The research showed that as long as the volunteers kept up their juggling practice these brain changes were also maintained, but when they stopped rehearsing their new skill their occipital lobes reverted back to their pre-juggling state. The findings from the juggling study also suggest that learning a new skill, even one that appears quite niche and specialized, may be an asset in other situations. For example, if learning to juggle increases your ability to rapidly identify and pick out objects in space so that you can react appropriately, juggling may make you a better and safer driver.

How can neuroplasticity change your life?

Once you realize just how adaptable your brain is, you can

Neuroplasticity Of The Brain

begin to appreciate the potential it has to change your life! Thanks to your brain"s plasticity, you can learn new skills, and change your attitude and outlook. Just think how much more productive you could become at work if you rewired your brain for greater focus, or imagine how much happier you could be if you trained it to think happier thoughts! The following chapters will tell you exactly how to improve every area of your life using practical, easy-to-use exercises.

Laying the groundwork – diet and sleep

As you have already seen, your choices and behaviors play a significant role in shaping your brain and your capabilities. However, in order to give your brain the best possible chance to forge new neuronal networks it is important to take good care of your physical health. You should therefore aim to make your lifestyle as healthy as possible. A healthy brain is a plastic brain that is receptive to new experiences.

Firstly, it is important to get enough sleep. It sounds so simple and obvious, yet most Western adults do not get the 6-8 hours per night recommended by most health experts. Whilst it is true that some people need more sleep than others, chances are that 8 hours per night is a good starting point. You can always cut back on the amount of time you spend in bed if you can function well with less. Staying up late might seem like a good way of maximizing your time and getting more work done, but it can backfire. A chronic lack of sleep results in lowered concentration levels, higher amounts of stress hormones, diminished ability to focus, and increased difficulty in making decisions.

Exercise: Schedule Your Sleep

Take a close look at your sleeping space. Is your bed

comfortable? Is your bedroom free of distractions? When you turn the lights out at night, is your bedroom truly dark enough to ensure that you get a good night's rest? If you find it difficult to relax at night, try creating a bedtime routine that prepares you for sleep. Depending on your personality and preferences, this may include activities such as meditation (more on this later in the book), having a warm bath, reading a few pages of an uplifting book, cuddling with a partner or pet, writing in a journal, or taking a few moments to think about what went well that day.

Diet is another important consideration when you are trying to optimize your brain function. In order to maintain healthy connections between neurons, your body needs an ongoing supply of omega-3 fatty acids. These can be found in oily fish, soybeans, walnuts, flaxseeds, spinach and chia seeds. Aim to eat 2-3 portions of oily fish such as mackerel each week, and add in the other foods mentioned above as often as you can.

Antioxidants are also vital in maintaining brain health. These compounds are found predominantly in fruits and vegetables. They are beneficial to the brain because they buffer it against oxidative stress, a natural reaction that occurs in response to your cells interacting with oxygen and releasing molecules known as "free radicals" which can trigger cell damage. Oxidative stress also happens as the result of interactions with pollutants and harmful chemicals, with smoking, alcohol and air pollution being common causes. Fortunately, antioxidants can reduce the overall impact of this phenomenon. Make sure you eat at least 5 portions of fruit and vegetables every day. They should be raw or steamed rather than boiled or fried, as harsh methods of cooking can drastically lower the antioxidant content.

Exercise: Make A Brain Food Shopping List

Think about what you eat in a typical day. Do you get enough omega-3 fatty acids and antioxidants? If not, how could you incorporate them into your diet on a more frequent basis? Simple changes such as scattering berries over your breakfast cereal or swapping red meat for oily fish one night of the week could go a long way in safeguarding the neuroplasticity of your brain.

Chapter 2: Overhaul Your Attitude and Shape a More Positive Mind

Having read the previous chapter, you now know that thanks to the pliable nature of your brain, you have the potential to learn new skills. In Chapter 3, we will take this idea further and look at some practical steps you can take to help you maximize your intellectual ability. However, neuroplasticity isn"t just useful in improving your vocabulary or learning to play a musical instrument. It"s also your passport to the development of new life skills and a whole new outlook on life in general. In this chapter, you will come to understand how your brain"s malleability is an enormous asset when it comes to making changes in your approach to life.

Positive thinking is a skill

You may believe that some people are simply born positive thinkers, and that this element of a person"s character is largely fixed. Whilst it is true that there is a heritable component to personality traits, there is increasing evidence that if you are willing to put in the effort to change your thinking patterns, both your brain and behaviors will help move you in a more positive direction. People who have mastered the art of positive thinking are more likely to be successful in all areas of their life. Note that being a positive thinker does not mean that you wilfully discount constructive criticism or refuse to face up to reality. Instead, it simply means that you are willing to believe in yourself and the possibility that most situations contain at least the potential seeds of a good outcome. Just as driving around London repeatedly helps develop neural networks in taxi drivers responsible for successful spatial navigation, repeated practice at positive thinking helps you automatically search for the upsides whenever you hit a roadblock in life. This ultimately helps you build resilience, which is protective against depression and helps you overcome the challenges life throws at you.

Depression, neuroplasticity, and the practice of positive thought

The effects of depression on the brain have been invaluable in developing our understanding of neuroplasticity and how it relates to mood and cognitive function. Recent research has demonstrated that depression is not just a mental state or experience, but a neurological event that has far-reaching consequences beyond a feeling of being "down" or "sad." Depression is a mental illness characterised by a number of psychological, emotional and physical symptoms including feelings of sadness, feelings of hopelessness, thoughts of death or suicide, loss of interest in previously-enjoyed activities, changes in weight and appetite, vague or random aches and pains with no discernible physical cause, and a tendency to withdraw from social situations.

Psychologists believe that there are several underlying factors that may cause or at least contribute to depression, including genetic predisposition and neurochemical imbalance. Some of these may be beyond your conscious control. On the other hand, there is also plenty of evidence to suggest that a significant factor that keeps depression going is an individual"s thinking style. Put simply, people who suffer from depression tend to see the world in a maladaptive way that keeps them locked in a cycle of negative thinking, negative actions, and withdrawal from the world around them. To break the feelings of bleak pessimism that often accompany depression and keep it going, it"s important that a depressed person retrains their brain to interpret external events in a more constructive way.

This is the rationale behind a type of psychotherapy known as Cognitive Behavioral Therapy, or CBT. The principle of CBT is as follows: It isn"t just what happens to us in life that can make us feel a particular way – what ultimately determines how we feel is the meaning we personally ascribe to external events. CBT practitioners believe that a key difference separating those with depression from those who are mentally healthy is that the former group habitually fall back on negative ways of viewing the world. In other words, when you are depressed, you continually teach yourself that the world is a bad place, that you will get hurt on a regular basis, and that there is little reason to think that things will get better. This style of thinking becomes "normal," and over time you may not even realize just how deeply your pessimistic your thinking style has become entrenched.

By now, you know that neurons firing together tend to wire together. Think negative thoughts on a regular basis and they will come to represent your reality. This has discernible effects on the brain. Studies comparing the brains of people with and without depression have found that mental illness can induce a state of "negative neuroplasticity" in which certain thinking and behavioral patterns become entrenched and maintain the symptoms. Research carried out at the University of Michigan using a brain scanning method known as positron emission tomography (PET) found that people with untreated depression have significantly fewer serotonin receptors than those not diagnosed with the condition. This is important because in order to feel happy and regulate our moods, our brains need to be able to make proper use of this neurotransmitter.

Other findings have revealed that depressed people tend to experience shrinkage of the hippocampus, which in turn leaves them vulnerable to problems in mood regulation and reduced memory function. The more episodes of depression an individual suffers, the greater the extent of the hippocampal damage. Given that depression is a risk factor for the development of Alzheimer"s disease, and that the hippocampus is among the first parts of the brain to be damaged in patients with this condition, it seems likely that the key to this link is an impaired hippocampus. More research is needed in this area, the takeaway message here is simply that depression changes the human brain. Fortunately, there is also plenty of evidence that psychotherapy, in which people suffering from depression are taught new ways of seeing the world and to challenge their negative thoughts, is an effective treatment. Even if you have been depressed or prone to negative thinking for many years, there is reason for hope – our brains never lose their plasticity, so with the right intervention and behavioral change, you can reverse the damage.

Exercise: Challenging Negative Thoughts

Whilst negative thought patterns are especially common in depression, most of us feel their effects from time to time. If you allow them too much mental airtime, however, you can begin to feel your attitude towards others and life in general become less optimistic. This can have a destructive effect on your everyday behavior. This exercise is often used by CBT therapists.

1. Identify a negative thought that you find yourself thinking on a frequent basis. This may relate to your social situation (e.g. "I have no friends"), your self-image ("I'm so incompetent and can't do anything") or about the world in general ("Everyone is so selfish and only out for what they can get"). Write it down and rate its believability on a scale of 1-10, with 10 indicating that you accept this thought as being absolutely true.
2. Now it's time to play detective. What evidence do you

have that this thought is actually true? Write down your evidence in favor of this thought. Now look at it from another angle – if you were to present the other side of the case, what evidence could you put forward in support of the motion that this perspective simply isn't true? For example, if you wrote down "I'm so incompetent and can't do anything" in Step 1, it's time to acknowledge that whilst you may not be as proficient in a certain field as you would like, you have succeeded in various other areas and have mastered other skills.

3. Once you have reviewed the evidence, re-evaluate how far you accept your negative thought as being an accurate reflection of reality. If you have taken the time to generate evidence for both sides (i.e. the statement being true and untrue), you should find that its power over you has been lessened.

4. As an additional step, think about whether or not your negative thought is actually helpful. Even supposing it is completely true (which is unlikely), what do you gain from holding onto it as though it were valid? Destructive thought patterns seldom inspire positive change. Consider the benefits of giving yourself permission to think differently.

This exercise is effective because it forces you to realize that the world is not black and white, and that even your most cherished negative beliefs are not immune to the power of critical thinking! If you repeat this exercise whenever you feel yourself slipping into negative thoughts, you will soon train yourself to challenge negativity rather than tolerating it or accepting it as your "normal state."

From now on, promise yourself that you are not going to sit back and accept the unnecessary negativity that your brain throws at you. Instead, pledge to see unhelpful negative thoughts as bad mental habits that you can correct with patience and effort. Some people find that keeping a journal helps them identify and tackle negative thinking. It isn"t realistic to try and write down every negative thought that crosses your mind, but you can certainly make use of your journal in noting down particular themes and devising alternatives to recurrent negative thoughts. Journaling is much easier to stick to when you make it a habit. Remember, when you repeat an action many times, your brain will come to expect it and you will feel uncomfortable if you deviate from your routine. You probably brush your teeth every morning and evening without having to think about it.

That"s because you have repeated the same action hundreds of times before. The same can become true of journaling or any other new habit that you want to instil. Set a time and place for your journaling practice and commit to it for 30 days. We"ll come back to goal-setting and habits in Chapter 4.

Why "Fake it „til you make it" really works – the Facial Feedback Hypothesis

The old cliché of "Fake it „til you make it!" may sound trite and unhelpful if you feel down, but psychologists have discovered that this phrase has merit. Most of us think that our emotions and body language are related as follows: We experience an event or memory, a particular emotion is triggered within us, and our body language changes as a result. We smile when we are happy, sit slumped in our chairs when we are feeling despondent, and so on. Whilst this is true, did you know that there is plenty of research showing that it also works the other way around? You smile because you are happy, but if you make a conscious decision to smile despite feeling grumpy or low, you are likely to feel a genuine uptick in your mood. This phenomenon, whereby the brain receives feedback from facial expressions and other forms of body language in such a way that the individual actually feels their mood or attitude shift, is known as the Facial Feedback Hypothesis. Early studies in this area used volunteers who were asked to hold a pencil between their teeth as they looked at cartoon strips. Those who were asked to hold a pencil horizontally between their teeth rated the cartoons as being funnier than the volunteers who were asked to hold a pencil in such a way that did not force their lips into a smile. The researchers concluded that because the horizontal-pencil group were in effect made to adopt a

"happy" expression, their brains interpreted the cartoons as especially amusing. Other studies have shown that adopting "power poses" (such as standing with your legs apart, back straight and with your hands on your hips) is a genuine confidence-booster in nerve-wracking situations. These findings are exciting because they imply that we already have the neural pathways in place that allow our brains to associate certain gestures, facial expressions and posture with particular mood states. Why not take advantage of these inbuilt circuits?

Exercise: Try the Facial Feedback Hypothesis For Yourself

The more often you encourage yourself to adopt positive body language, the more natural it will feel, and the more you will strengthen the link between physical movement and your mental state. Getting into the habit of sitting up straight and smiling, even when you don't feel like it, will mean that you have ready access to a quick mood boost wherever you are. So the next time you need a pick-me-up, put the Facial Feedback Hypothesis into action.

Mindfulness and its effects on the brain

Over the past decade, "mindfulness" has become a common buzzword in psychology and psychiatry circles. However, it has proven itself to be more than a passing fad. It turns out that practicing mindfulness results in changes to the brain that can help you feel less stressed, maintain a healthy perspective on events in your life, and reduce your susceptibility to depression. Mindfulness also enables you to make better decisions, which holds exciting implications for those working in a number of fields including crime prevention, education, and social work.

What exactly does "mindfulness" mean? At its most basic, mindfulness is simply the act of focusing your attention on the present moment. It means being willing to stop worrying about the future or ruminate about past events. When you behave mindfully, you are living with full awareness of where and who you are right now. You can practice mindfulness anywhere.

Exercise: Mindful Washing Up

When you next need to wash a dish or spoon, take the opportunity to do a mindfulness exercise. As you run a bowl of soapy water, pay attention to the feel of the water on your skin, the scent of the washing-up liquid, and the sound it makes as it swirls around in the bowl. Feel the texture of the object you are washing against your fingertips. If you feel your attention wandering, notice that your focus has drifted before bringing it back gently but firmly to the present.

Mindfulness is often linked with meditation, a broad term that refers to the act of channeling your attention on a particular concept, object, or just your own breathing. Neither mindfulness nor meditation are exclusively the preserve of the religious. Although meditation is popularly linked with Buddhism and Hinduism, people of all faiths and none are able to benefit from practices that allow them mental breathing space.

How does neuroplasticity come into this equation? Studies with people who meditate regularly show that meditation literally shapes the human brain in such a way that enhances mood and wellbeing. For instance, a study published in the journal *Neuroreport* explained that compared with those who never meditated, people who practiced regularly tended to have thicker cortices. This was especially apparent in the areas of the cerebral cortex responsible for sensory processing and focused attention. (If you want to retain more of what you learn and focus for longer at school or work, meditation is a great way to improve your performance.)

Not only that, but long-term meditation also helps you exert more control over your emotions. This doesn"t mean that regular meditators turn into robots, just that meditation helps equip you with the power to keep strong emotions in check and make more conscious, controlled choices when it comes to responding to challenging situations.

Exercise: Mediation, Part I

Simple breathing meditation is a popular exercise for beginners. All you need to do is sit or stand in a comfortable position. Close your eyes and focus on your breathing. Count your breaths slowly. Keep all your attention focused on this once simple task. If your mind starts to drift, bring it back to your breath.

Exercise: Meditation, Part II

If you find it hard to sit still for any length of time or dislike focusing on your breath, walking meditation could be a great alternative. Pick a quiet room or area outside, and simply walk up and down in a straight line. Keep your walking pace even. Focus your attention on the sensation you can feel in your feet when they make contact with the ground.

Neuroplasticity Of The Brain

When you get into the habit of challenging your negative thoughts and meditating every day, you will soon find that your brain responds favorably to your new habits. Although you might not be able to see the changes on an MRI or PET scanner, you can be sure that your brain"s malleable nature will result in significant changes in your mood and overall outlook. Just think how much calmer and more pleasant life will be once you learn to exert greater control over your moods and emotional responses! Start by meditating for 2-3 minutes per day, then gradually build up to 20-30 minutes each morning or evening.

Andreas Senkbeil

Chapter 3: Enliven Your Learning

Is intelligence really fixed?

Until recently, most psychologists assumed that a person"s intelligence was fixed – that is, most believed that if you are smart, it"s because you were born that way. However, with the discovery that the human brain is plastic has come a shift in attitudes towards intelligence. Given that the source of our mental capabilities is the brain, you"ll be unsurprised to learn that with the right approach and a willingness to undertake exercises that help new neuronal connections form, you really can make yourself smarter.

How to boost your mental ability

The traditional view of IQ was that once you had reached adulthood, there is nothing you can do to improve your mental functioning. However, with the discovery that the brain is plastic comes an important implication – you can work on your cognitive abilities and problem-solving skills. When it comes to forging and maintaining connections between neurons, the old adage of "use it or lose it" is true. It doesn"t matter whether you are 8, 18 or 88 – through repeated effort and a commitment to improving your mental abilities, you can sharpen your mental prowess. In fact, just by learning that intelligence is fluid, you have already taken the first step. Researchers from Stanford and Columbia have discovered that students are more likely to feel positive about their studies and achieve higher grades if they are taught that they can improve their own intelligence. This is because when you shift your mindset around mental ability, you leave yourself open to developing new skills. Your motivation also increases, because whenever you hit a roadblock or simply don"t feel like continuing with a particular activity, you can hold the outcome in mind and know that with sufficient application you can and will achieve your goal of improving your skills.

If you were told in school that you weren"t especially smart or capable, you need to work on discarding these unhelpful beliefs. Remind yourself that only in the past couple of decades has neuroplasticity become an accepted fact within mainstream science, and even today there is still a widespread belief that intellectual ability is predetermined at birth.

Adopt a growth mindset

"Growth mindset" refers to the attitude that it is possible to shape your intelligence with nothing more than your own determination and actions. It also involves taking a balanced, realistic view of how people learn. This includes adjusting your attitude towards perfectionism. Too often, we can fall into the trap of feeling that unless we can master a skill perfectly and in a short timeframe, it isn"t worth trying in the first place. This way of thinking is destructive for a couple of reasons. For a start, placing yourself under such a high level of pressure will cause you unnecessary stress, which is not conducive to productive learning. When you are preoccupied with making negative judgements about your own capabilities and putting yourself down, you are not in a position to concentrate and learn.

Second, it is essential that if you want to learn and grow that you become comfortable with failure and setbacks. This is because only at the limits of your intellectual comfort zone do you have the opportunity to mentally stretch yourself. Feedback – both positive and negative – allows you the chance to understand your strengths and weaknesses in order to make progress. People who see intelligence as fixed find failure threatening, because they interpret it as evidence that they might not be as smart as they would like to believe. On the other hand, if you acknowledge that neuroplasticity means that intellectual ability is malleable and that sustained effort results in change, you can afford to see failure as just another step on your learning journey. Once you make this mental shift, you stop frittering your time away on berating yourself and instead channel that energy into figuring out new strategies by which you can improve your skills and development. In addition, you will become less bothered by criticism. You will realize that even if someone is correct when they say you aren"t especially good at a particular skill, this doesn"t mean you cannot improve in the future. Neither does it mean that you aren"t capable in other domains. With a growth mindset, you stop seeing intelligence as an all-or-nothing entity and more a collection of abilities that you can develop with the right application.

Another benefit of a growth mindset is that you will feel less threatened by other peoples" success. If you see intelligence as something that only some people possess, you will feel as though you are in competition with others. However, when you understand that everyone has a flexible level of intelligence and is at a different stage in their personal journeys, you will find other peoples" successes inspirational.

Exercise: Developing A Growth Mindset

Just like any other mental habit, it takes time to adopt a growth mindset. Take the time to examine your self-limiting beliefs around intelligence and your own capabilities. Ask yourself the following questions:

When you think back to your school days, do you remember being made to feel clever, stupid, or somewhere in between?

When you think of taking up a new skill, what thoughts run through your mind?

Do you know how you learn best? For example, are you more likely to learn by reading, watching, hearing, making, or via another medium?

There are no "right" or "wrong" answers to these questions, and you don't have to show your answers to anyone else. These prompts are designed to help you reflect on your current approach to learning. Don't worry if you discover that your own beliefs are holding you back – when you have internalized the key messages within this book and started to prove for yourself the power of neuroplasticity and habit change, they will begin to change!

Exercise: Learn How To Change Your Relationship To Failure

Continue to cultivate a growth mindset by re-examining your relationship to failure. Think of a time you came up against an obstacle when learning a new skill. For example, you may have failed an exam in the past. Looking at the situation from a growth mindset, how could you have learned from this experience? Now that you know how plastic your brain is and how much potential you have when it comes to future learning, you can take a step backwards, detach emotionally and take a pragmatic approach. For example, could you have sought feedback on your exam answers and then re-taken the test? Could you have chosen to see the experience as a starting point for rethinking your learning and revision strategies?

IQ versus everyday skills

The most famous measure of intelligence is the

Intelligence Quotient, more commonly referred to as "IQ."

Although it is usually presented as a single figure, your IQ is actually comprised of a number of skills such as verbal reasoning (the ability to use, communicate with and understand words) and mathematical capacity. This means that whilst it may be fun and rewarding to try and raise your IQ score, it"s more helpful to focus on Although you don"t need to know your IQ or fixate on attaining a certain number, it"s encouraging to note that psychologists have long known that IQ is malleable. In the 1990s, New Zealand researcher James Flynn took a careful look at IQ scores obtained from populations around the world. He noticed that every generation from the 1930s onwards appeared to outdo their parents on measures of

IQ. This phenomenon was labelled the "Flynn Effect" by authors Richard Herrnstein and Charles Murray in their book *The Bell Curve*, published in 1994.

Exercise: Hone In On The Skills You Want To Improve

If you are reading this chapter, chances are that you want to become "smarter." That's a good starting point, but if you want to make tangible progress you need to locate your weaknesses and then come up with a plan of action that will allow you to improve. Make a list of intellectual skills you want to develop, and things you would like to learn about. Add as much detail as possible. For example, your list may resemble the following:

- Learn how to speak French to an intermediate level
- Learn how to carry out mental arithmetic
- Learn how to draw 3D objects

Once you have set down what you want to learn in black and white, you will realize that "smart" actually comes in many flavors, and it's up to you to decide where you want to focus your attention.

Whatever you want to learn, you must practice

There is no magic secret to maximizing your brainpower – that"s the bad news. The good news is that the path to greater success is simple. You just need to decide exactly what you want to learn, how best to learn it, and then put in the hours required. The three steps to bear in mind are "Repeat," "Retrieve," and "Review."

You need to embrace repetition, because this is what will solidify the neural networks in your brain. Think of your neural networks as being like tracks across a muddy field. When a track is used repeatedly, it becomes deeper and further engrained into the ground. Anyone using it regularly will be able to drive across the field faster and faster as time goes on and the track becomes deeper. In a similar way, the more you practice or revisit a skill or area of knowledge, the more deeply entrenched your learning will become.

However, simple repetition – such as reading the same book over and over again or playing the same pieces on the violin for several weeks in a row – is worthless without meaningful engagement and variety. Specifically, passive repetition isn"t sufficiently attention-grabbing or challenging enough to make an appreciable difference to your neural networks. Try to

approach material in a number of ways. Mind maps and quizzes are two useful tools that can make repetition more effective.

Exercise: Make A Mind Map

Andreas Senkbeil

In order to make as many new neural connections as possible, you need to train your brain to draw associations between diverse concepts. Making a mind map is a great way of doing this, because it allows you to experiment with potential links between various topics. This method works best if you are attempting to learn a great deal of detailed information on a specific topic. Begin by placing the central idea or title in the middle of a large piece of paper. Now write relevant sub-headings or key facts on smaller pieces of paper or sticky notes. Now comes the fun part – how can you best arrange them in a way that connects them all together? Play around with concepts and see how they fit to make a coherent whole or "big picture." Draw lines, arrows and annotations as appropriate.

For example, if you have an interest in mental health and wanted to brush up on your knowledge of common mental illnesses, your mind map may feature "MENTAL ILLNESSES" written in the center, with sub-topics such as "Depression" and "Anxiety" written on sticky notes dotted around the page. You might then realize, as you consider what you have learned on both topics, that the two share a few similar symptoms and are frequently seen together in the same patient. You might then decide to draw a line between the two and write "ARE SIMILAR" to illustrate your point.

Once you feel as though you have absorbed or learned some new information or picked up a skill, the next step is to practice retrieval. In other words – test yourself! Testing yourself is a way of checking just how deep the metaphorical muddy tracks go. When you can readily retrieve informat ion, it"s a sure sign that you are making the most of your plastic brain and laying down some new neural circuits.

Quizzes and tests are a great way of testing out your new knowledge, whether theoretical or practical. There are plenty of quiz books and study guides available on almost every subject you could think of, but quizzes and tests are even more effective when you devise them yourself. This is because the very act of setting yourself a challenge or writing the quiz questions forces you to engage once more with the material, which serves to further reinforce the new circuits you are laying down. Furthermore, you will also gain a sense of accomplishment when you create a set of questions because doing so requires thought and creativity.

Exercise: Create Your Own Quiz

Take a stack of index cards. On one side of each card, write a question. On the other side, write the answer along with a short explanation if appropriate. Mix the question formats up to maintain your interest. For example, include multiple choice, open-ended, definition-based and true/false questions in your question card pack. Shuffle the cards and then set them down in a pile. You can test yourself or ask someone else to read you each question. If you answer a question correctly, set it to one side. If you answer incorrectly, keep the card in the deck. Your objective is to answer every question correctly, even if it means posing the same question on several occasions!

Explaining a concept to someone else also serves the dual purposes of repetition and retrieval. Ask a patient friend or relative whether you could give them an oral presentation on a particular topic. If they can listen attentively and then ask probing questions that force you to repeat and re-process the information in a new way, then so much the better!

Review

The more enjoyment you can derive from learning, the more likely you are to practice and in turn to make progress.

Stepping beyond your current level of expertise

Always seek to challenge yourself. As we have already established, to learn a new skill you must be willing to repeat the same behavior over and over again. However, to become truly proficient and perform at a high level, you must also be willing to risk failure and defeat by attempting to push yourself further and further. For example, suppose you want to become an accomplished violinist. To do this, it is essential to practice playing the violin at frequent intervals. However, it is not enough to play the same pieces over and over again, as this will limit the extent to which you can make progress. You need to continually make the effort to go one step beyond your competence level. This is why having a tutor or learning with other people can be so effective – they can serve to shake you free of complacency and encourage you to

Learning needs context to be most effective

Remember that a central principle of neuroplasticity is that pre-existing neural networks become stronger the more frequently they are activated. This means that putting new knowledge and skills into pre-existing contexts. For example, suppose you are learning French and are working on expanding your vocabulary and grammar. To help cement your learning and put your language circuits into practice, try using new words and grammatical principles alongside those you already know. If you were learning about a period in history, say for an upcoming assignment or test in college, you may remember the details more readily if you put that particular time period in context with events that came before and after it.

Learn how to read more quickly

If you are currently studying for a qualification, or you are just serious about learning a lot of new information for your own personal benefit, assess your reading speed. Most adults read between 250 and 300 words per minute. With practice, however, it is possible to obtain reading speeds of up to 800 words per minute! Think of how much more information you will be able to pick up in a short amount of time if you train your brain to absorb written detail at a rapid rate. There are many good books and guides out there on speed reading, but the following exercise will get you started.

Exercise: Start Learning To Speed Read

A popular exercise for those learning to speed read involves utilizing a pointer. Find a book that you would like to read. Time how long it takes you to read a page when you read in your usual manner. Now take a sharpened pencil and position it so that the lead is directly under the first word on a new page. Repeat the exercise but this time, move your pointer along as you read. You should find that your reading speed accelerates. This is because you are helping your eyes and brain to focus directly on the material rather than jumping all over the page, as weaker readers tend to do. With practice, you will no longer need the pointer because your malleable brain will have been trained to read more efficiently.

Don"t overlook emotional intelligence – boost your EQ and social intelligence

Increasingly, psychologists recognize not only the value of traditional intelligence but also the merits of emotional intelligence, sometimes referred to as EQ. An emotionally intelligent person is good at detecting and managing emotions in others. They can rely on themselves not to let their emotions override their good judgement, and they are good at communicating their wants and needs. If you practice the exercises suggested in the previous chapter, you will naturally become more emotionally and socially intelligent because your perspective on the world will be realistic but positive and you will be well-placed to deal with your reactions and those of other people. This will also make you socially intelligent – you will be able to pick up on how other people are feeling, and be suitably assertive in how you strike a balance between their needs and your own. Try the exercise below and train yourself in a key skill in social intelligence – reading body language.

Exercise: Train Yourself To Be A Body Language Expert

For ten minutes every day, put your TV on mute and flick through the channels until you find a drama or soap opera in which two or three people are engaged in conversation or conflict. Watch the characters interact, paying attention to their body language. What is the dynamic between the characters? How are they feeling?

Once you have "read" them, turn the sound back on. Was your assessment accurate? Doing this exercise on a regular basis allows you to train yourself in the art of understanding body language. This can have a positive effect on your social life and your ability to create rapport with other people, as they will feel as though you understand them.

Consider learning to play a musical instrument

Research suggests that when you learn to read music and practice playing an instrument on a regular basis, you increase your mental capacities beyond just being able to distinguish between a treble and bass clef or how to place your fingers at the right angle on an oboe. Amongst other skills, becoming a musician improves your attention span and memory. The implications are clear – growing your cognitive capacities in these domains has a highly beneficial effect on your abilities in other areas. Whatever you are trying to learn, being able to pay attention to new information and stimuli and being able to remember is a definite advantage.

Exercise: Become A Musician

If you do not already play a musical instrument on a regular basis, aim to try some music lessons over the coming month. Pick an instrument you have always wanted to try, and look up a local music teacher. Most instruments can be hired on a monthly basis from a music shop or online service whilst you see whether it suits you.

When you implement the exercises in this chapter, you will soon notice that your learning becomes more efficient. You will feel smarter, and pick up new skills and knowledge more readily. Remember that your brain is your best asset and has huge potential. Start employing it today!

Chapter 4: Go for Your Goals

Now that you understand the basics mechanisms of neuroplasticity and what your brain can achieve with the right training, it"s time to put your knowledge to good use and start setting some goals! Given that you chose and downloaded this book, you are likely to be at a point in your life whereby you want to make some real and lasting changes. In this chapter, you will learn how to visualize your desired outcomes, and why this will improve your chances of success. You will learn how to overcome your bad habits and replace them with positive behaviors. You will set your personal goals based on SMART criteria, and give yourself the best possible chance of building the habits and patterns that will help you make progress in any area of your life.

The value of visualization

You may have heard that many professional athletes, actors and public speakers use visualization before giving a performance. This involves imagining the desired outcome in as much detail as possible. For example, a competitive swimmer may imagine themselves starting the race with a strong movement from the side of the pool, maintaining a steady pace, remaining ahead of the other competitors and reaching the finishing line first.

Why does visualization work? Basically, when you imagine undertaking a particular activity, your brain reacts as though it is really happening. Natan Sharansky, a man kept in solitary confinement for 9 years in a USSR prison, decided that to make good use of his time on the inside. To stop himself from going mad he would practice chess moves. However, as he was not allowed a chess set, he had to play each game in his head. After his release from jail, he managed to triumph over world chess champion Garry Kasparov. Sharansky had trained his brain using nothing more than regular visualization and mental practice. Even more remarkably, mental visualization can actually increase muscle mass! Ohio-based psychologist Guang Ye carried out a study in which he compared changes in muscle development in people who went to the gym for regular workouts with those who only imagined undertaking exercise. As you might expect, the participants who went to the gym increased their strength significantly, by an average of 30%. However, those who simply sat and imagined working out and lifting weights still increased their performance by 13.5%. Therefore, we know that directed visualization has a tangible effect on the body that extends beyond brain cells.

Exercise: Visualize Your Outcome
If you want to improve your performance in any particular situation, visualization is a great place to start. For example, perhaps you want to feel more confident when giving a speech. In this case, you would imagine yourself remaining calm backstage, and perceiving the butterflies in your stomach as pleasant anticipation rather than fear. You would then imagine yourself taking your position at the podium before delivering your speech in a clear, assertive tone of voice. Whatever you are visualizing, be sure to employ all of your senses as you imagine your desired outcome. What do you see, hear, smell, taste, touch and feel in your imagined scenario?

You can use visualization every day in the run-up to a specific event, as performers do, or you can use it to cement your commitment to particular goals. For example, you may set yourself the goal of starting your own business within a year. In this case, you could dedicate several minutes every day to visualizing how you will feel and what you will experience when you sit down in the morning at your desk (or wherever your place of work might be) to begin another day of working for yourself. If you want to become more comfortable in social settings, you may set yourself the goal of attending two social events each week. In this case, you could use visualization to conjure up an image of you navigating a social setting with comfort and confidence, making conversation and laughing with those around you.

The SMART goals checklist

Whether you want to begin a new business venture, overhaul your garden or write that novel, SMART goals are the best way of setting yourself up for success. When devising a goal, make sure that it meets the following criteria:

Specific: Get precise with what you want. For example, "I will lose 10lbs" is a specific goal, whereas "I will lose some weight" is not.

Measurable: You should have a means of assessing whether you have truly met your target. Otherwise, how will you know whether you have succeeded?

Achievable: It"s great to set ambitious goals, but make sure that you actually stand a chance of meeting your goals! Otherwise you will become demoralized.

Relevant: Each goal should represent a step closer to where you want to be. For example, if you want to cut down on your drinking, setting a goal to eat less junk food might be somewhat related (both intentions set you up for a healthier lifestyle), but it isn"t relevant to your ultimate goal.

Time bound: Your goal should have an endpoint. For instance, "I will quit smoking within 3 months" is a time bound goal, whereas "I will quit smoking soon" is not.

Exercise: Set Three SMART Goals

Take a piece of paper and a pen and write down three goals you want to achieve over the coming year. Are they SMART goals? If not, reword them until they meet each of the criteria above. If you feel overwhelmed by a large goal, set smaller sub-goals instead. Now start visualizing your ideal outcomes and making your first steps today!

Setting goals to break bad habits

Have you been trying to give up a bad habit for many years? Now that you can appreciate the power of habit and how easy it is to train your brain to act in maladaptive ways, you can take steps to overcome them! It doesn"t matter how many times you have indulged in your habits over the years – with a bit of determination and the right approach, you can overhaul your routine and feel better for it.

Exercise: Plan To Rewire A Bad Habit

Pick a habit you want to overcome and take a close look at it. What are the typical triggers for this behavior? Once you start to unpick the context, you stand a better chance of devising alternative behaviors that benefit you. Your task is to identify the conditions surrounding each habit, and then come up with new behaviors that you can repeat on a regular basis. For instance, suppose you want to give up the habit of buying a chocolate bar on the way home from work every evening. Let's say that when you consider the problem carefully, a number of associations and behaviors combine to keep this habit going – you leave work at a particular time, you walk down a particular road, you go into a particular shop, and so on. Now, what could you do to break the chain? Perhaps you could get into the habit of walking a new route home? Get creative and then commit to implementing the habit of breaking the chain for 30 days in a row.

It can be difficult and frustrating to try and break bad habits. On the other hand, you now know that there are grounds for optimism – given that our brains are sufficiently plastic that we can develop bad habits, they are also plastic enough that we can adopt new and healthier behaviors! Set sensible goals, break habit chains, visualize better outcomes and repeat new behaviors – these steps really work and let you harness your brain"s malleability.

Why you should consider finding an accountability partner

An accountability partner can be of great help when it comes to goal-setting and personal development. If you have a relative or friend who has expressed interest in any of the concepts in this book, ask them whether they would be interested in becoming your accountability buddy. This means that the two of you agree on a schedule by which you "check in" with one another on a fortnightly, weekly or perhaps even daily basis. For instance, if you are trying to give up eating junk food using some of the principles and exercises in this book, you could ask your accountability buddy to call you a couple of times a week to get an honest summary of your diet over the previous few days. If you both want to work on the same goal, you could even set up a regular day and time for carrying out a particular activity. For example, if you are both interested in meditation, then you could agree to attend the same class each week plus hold one another accountable to a private thirty-minute meditation session every morning. Being able to talk to one another about the difficulties of breaking bad habits and thinking about life in a new way can be very encouraging.

The role of rewards in meeting goals

Good old-fashioned rewards and ethical bribes can also be an effective way of encouraging change. You could use any of the free or low-cost goal tracker apps out there, or take a more traditional tack and create a progress chart or graph using old-fashioned pen and paper. Choose suitable rewards that encourage your new, healthy habits. For instance, don"t reward a week of snack-free living with a large bar of chocolate! You should also make sure that when you promise yourself a reward, that you get it. Otherwise, you are teaching yourself that you cannot be relied upon to deliver your own promises. Once you choose a reward or outcome, stick by your intentions.

Exercise: Create A Reward Board

This exercise makes use of two useful concepts in goal setting – visualization and rewards. For each goal, take a large piece of cardboard or a corkboard. Now find slogans and images that capture or represent your ideal outcome. For instance, if your goal is to save a certain sum of money and put down a deposit on a house, you could include images of the kind of house you want to buy, together with paint or fabric swatches. Keep the board where you can see it. This will help you to literally keep your end goal in mind, which in turn will reinforce your motivation. As the old saying goes, keep your eyes on the prize!

How to reinforce your new changes

Another useful technique in changing your self-image and increasing the likelihood that you will reach your goals is via affirmations. Affirmations are short, incisive statements that tie in nicely with visualization. They work by encouraging you to believe and act as though you have already attained a particular goal or outcome, or are at least making progress in the right direction. A few examples show how this works in practice.

Let"s say that your goal is to lose weight, and in doing so both improve your diet and increase the amount of exercise you get every week. Examples of suitable affirmations in this case may include:

"I am getting slimmer every day."
"I am becoming healthier and I love it."
"As time goes on, I look and feel better and better."
"I enjoy eating healthy food and taking regular exercise." "I am succeeding in meeting my weight loss goal."

Note that good affirmations have the following properties in common. Firstly, they should be directly related to the goal or outcome you are trying to achieve. Secondly, they should be positive. There is no room for indecisive language, self-doubt or ambiguity when it comes to writing successful affirmations. Just saying them out loud should make you feel fired up with positive energy and a renewed belief in yourself and your goals! Third, a good affirmation should be brief and memorable. There is no point in creating long-winded statements that you won"t be able to memorize.

Affirmations work on the brain in the same way as visualization exercises. When you repeat an intention or outcome to yourself on a regular basis, your brain starts to accept this state of affairs as reality. This triggers a cascade effect whereby your behaviors begin to reflect your new beliefs. A virtuous cycle begins in which you accept your affirmations, act in line with your new beliefs, gain evidence that you are capable of change, are even more likely to behave in more adaptive ways, and so on.

Exercise: Devise Your Own Affirmations

Based on the checklist above, put together at least three affirmations of your own that relate to your goals and desires. Now find a way of incorporating them into your everyday life. Some people like to repeat their affirmations when they wake up in the morning, to provide a positive beginning to their day. Others like to say them last thing at night. Experiment and find out what works best for you.

If you have adopted meditation as a regular practice, you can combine it with affirmations and visualization for an effective lift whenever you feel as though you have hit a slump when it comes to making headway with your goals. For instance, suppose that you come up against an obstacle in your weight loss journey – you go on vacation and gain a couple of pounds. The best way to handle such a setback is not to bully yourself or fall into self-pity, but to use positive self-talk and affirmations to get things back on track.

To continue with this particular example, you could set aside half an hour to re-center yourself and recommit to your weight loss goal. Beginning with 15 minutes of meditation would allow you to re-connect with your body and ground yourself in the present, which in turn would help you stop mentally beating yourself up for a lapse. You could then spend several minutes using visualization techniques, thinking about how you will resume your diet and exercise plan with immediate effect. You could imagine how good you will look and feel after just a few weeks of following your plan, perhaps thinking about how great it will be to wake up in the morning full of energy or to go to the beach feeling confident in a swimsuit. Finally, you could then spend a few minutes using affirmations that reinforce the idea that you are doing well and will continue to make progress until you reach your desired outcome. Remember that taking a positive and proactive approach will get you much further in life than self-flagellation and rumination, whatever your goals and intentions might be. People rarely change as a result of criticism.

Conclusion: Where To Go From Here

You now have all the background knowledge you need to fully harness the power of neuroplasticity, together with plenty of practical exercises that will help you develop healthier habits, learn new ways of thinking, and train your brain so that you can move towards your most important life goals.

Remember that whilst your brain is plastic and has the potential to let you reach new heights of excellence, this won"t happen by itself! To get the most from your brain, you need to make an ongoing effort to change its wiring. That means being willing to implement the techniques outlined in this book on a regular basis. Neurons that fire together, wire together – so get firing them on a regular basis! For instance, meditation can yield immediate effects on your mood and calm you down quickly, but if you are serious about training your brain to help you make better decisions and live in the present on a daily basis rather than the past or the future, you need to make time in your life for practice. Set yourself relevant goals that will allow you to make steady progress. Make sure that these goals are challenging but achievable. You should be aiming to move beyond your comfort zone, but not so far that you become disheartened when you try and fail to meet a particular challenge. For example, it is not realistic to set yourself the goal of never again thinking a negative thought. On the other hand, it is feasible to set yourself the goal of devising challenges in the face of negative thinking at least five times every day. In this way, you are slowly setting yourself up to become a more positive thinker. You will soon get into the habit of confronting your bleakest thoughts with more constructive alternatives, and in doing so rewire your brain.

Andreas Senkbeil

Whatever your preferred approach to change and however you want to use your brain"s neuroplasticity, consistent practice is the key. Start changing your behaviors, thought patterns and life today. Good luck!

www.ingramcontent.com/pod-product-compliance
Lightning Source LLC
Chambersburg PA
CBHW070414190526
45169CB00003B/1252